The Diabetes etiquette:

Reduce and eliminate type 2 diabetes

By

Jesse R. Stewart

Table of Contents

Introduction

Diabetes has gone from being rare to being pandemic in only a generation, a disastrous shift that begs the pressing question: Why are so many people suffering, and so suddenly? And how, despite spending billions, have our health authorities been unable to provide an explanation or remedy for such a terrible scourge? Instead, they have characterized type 2 diabetes as a chronic, progressive condition that portends a life of slow, excruciating decline and early death. They have all but given up on finding a solution.

Tragically, diabetes experts from across the world have come to the conclusion that the best option for patients is to just control or delay the condition by relying on drugs, gadgets, and surgery for the rest of their lives. Better nutrition is not prioritized. As an alternative, some 45 worldwide medical and scientific institutions and associations decided in 2016 that bariatric surgery, which is costly and dangerous, should be the first line of therapy for diabetes. Another newly authorized proposal is a novel weight-loss technique that involves implanting a thin tube in the stomach to force food out of the body before all the calories can be absorbed. This surgery has been dubbed "medically approved bulimia" by some.

The revolutionary notion put out in these pages is that diabetes results from our systems' chronic overuse of carbs, which triggers an insulin response, and that cutting back on those carbohydrates is the healthiest and most natural method to treat the condition. A low-carbohydrate diet for the treatment of obesity is currently being used by hundreds of doctors around the world, and it is also supported by more than 75 clinical trials that involved thousands of participants and were conducted over an extended period of time, including several trials that lasted two years.

In order to go forward on a new road for the sake of truth, science, and greater health, we must embrace the reality of this book, start exploring the alternative science presented in this book, and accept it as a given.

Chapter 1

Diabetes as an epidemic

Diabetes is a chronic condition that arises when the pancreas does not create enough insulin or when the body does not utilize the insulin that is produced adequately. A hormone called insulin regulates blood sugar levels. Hyperglycemia, also known as elevated blood glucose or high blood sugar, is a common side effect of uncontrolled diabetes that can cause catastrophic damage to many of the body's systems, particularly the neurons and blood vessels, over time.

Diabetes affected 8.5% of persons aged 18 and above in 2014. Diabetes was the direct cause of 1.5 million fatalities in 2019, with 48% of all diabetes-related deaths occurring before the age of 70. Diabetes was responsible for another 460 000 renal disease fatalities, and elevated blood glucose is responsible for around 20% of cardiovascular mortality.

Diabetes caused a 3% rise in age-standardized death rates between 2000 and 2019. Diabetes-related mortality increased by 13% in lower-middle-income nations.

Between 2000 and 2019, the global risk of dying from any of the four major noncommunicable illnesses (cardiovascular diseases, cancer, chronic respiratory diseases, or diabetes) between the ages of 30 and 70 was reduced by 22%.

Key facts

• The number of persons living with diabetes increased from 108 million in 1980 to 422 million in 2014.

• Compared to high-income countries, prevalence has increased more quickly in low- and middle-income countries. Diabetes is a major factor in kidney failure, heart attacks, strokes, blindness, and lower limb amputation.

• Between 2000 and 2019, the age-specific mortality rates for diabetes rose by 3%.

• Diabetes and renal disease caused an estimated 2 million deaths in 2019.

•A nutritious diet, regular physical activity, keeping a normal body weight, and abstaining from tobacco use are all approaches to avoid or postpone the onset of type 2 diabetes.

• Diabetes may be treated and its repercussions prevented or postponed by diet, physical exercise, medication, and routine screening for complications.

Diabetes Symptoms

Diabetes symptoms might appear abruptly. Type 2 diabetes symptoms might be minor and may not be seen for many years.

Diabetes symptoms include:

- feeling very thirsty

- needing to pee more frequently than normal

- impaired vision

- feeling exhausted

Diabetes can cause damage to blood vessels in the heart, eyes, kidneys, and nerves over time.

Diabetes increases the risk of health complications such as heart attack, stroke, and kidney failure.

Diabetes can permanently impair eyesight by destroying blood vessels in the eyes.

As a result of nerve loss and insufficient blood flow, many diabetics experience foot issues. Amputation may be necessary as a result of foot ulcers caused by this.

Difference between Type 1 and Type 2 Diabetes

Type 1 (Idiopathic) Diabetes

Diabetes type 1 is characterized by insufficient insulin production and needs daily insulin treatment. Type 1 diabetes was formerly classified as insulin-dependent, juvenile, or childhood-onset. 9 million persons worldwide with type 1 diabetes as of 2017, with high-income nations housing the bulk of these individuals. We don't know what causes it or how to stop it.

Type 2 Diabetes

Your body's ability to utilize glucose (sugar) for energy is impacted by type 2 diabetes. It prevents the body from utilizing insulin effectively, which, if left untreated, can result in excessive blood sugar levels.

The body can suffer significant harm from type 2 diabetes over time, especially to the nerves and blood arteries.

Most cases of type 2 diabetes may be avoided. Being overweight, not getting enough exercise, and heredity all have a role in the development of type 2 diabetes.

The greatest symptoms of type 2 diabetes must be avoided by early detection. Regular check-ups and blood tests with a healthcare professional are the greatest methods to identify diabetes early.

Type 2 diabetes might have modest symptoms. It might be years before anyone notices them. Although frequently less severe, the symptoms of type 2 diabetes might be comparable to those of type 1. As a result, the ailment might not be identified until after it has caused issues.

Type 2 Diabetes affects more than 95% of those who have the disease. Previously known as adult-onset or non-insulin dependent type 2 Diabetes. This kind of diabetes was previously exclusively found in adults, but it is becoming increasingly common in kids as well.

LONG-TERM EFFECTS OF DIABETES ON THE BODY

Our bodies may suffer long-term effects from diabetes. Diabetic complications are a frequent phrase used to describe long-term harm.

Diabetes may affect every region of the body since it has an impact on our blood vessels and nerves.

However, certain areas of our bodies are more negatively impacted than others.

It often takes a number of years of poorly managed diabetes for diabetic complications to manifest. Maintaining strict control over your diabetes, blood pressure, and cholesterol will help you avoid complications and keep them away.

If you want to keep your blood sugar levels within the specified blood glucose level standards, you should follow a balanced diet, abstain from alcohol and tobacco, and get regular exercise into your daily routine.

Cardiovascular effects of diabetes

Coronary artery disease and diabetes have a strong connection.

Diabetes raises blood pressure and is associated with high cholesterol, both of which greatly increase the risk of heart attacks and cardiovascular disease.

Heart attacks and diabetes

High blood pressure and cholesterol increase the risk of strokes, much as diabetes has an impact on the heart.

Diabetes and its effects on the eyes

Diabetic retinopathy is a very frequent side effect of diabetes.

This illness is caused, like other complications, by a period of time with poorly managed or unmanaged diabetes. A multitude of symptoms are present in diabetic retinopathy.

Retinopathy is brought on by swollen and leaky blood vessels in the retina, which lines the back of the eye. Another risk factor for diabetic retinopathy is high blood pressure.

Since diabetic retinopathy is treatable, it is preferable to identify it as soon as possible. Attending a retinopathy screening appointment, which is offered free of charge on the NHS once a year, is the best method to do this.

Diabetes's impact on renal health

Diabetes, along with poorly managed diabetes, high blood pressure, and cholesterol, all raise the risk.

The term used to describe kidney damage brought on by diabetes is diabetic nephropathy.

Nephropathy screening can detect kidney damage early on since it develops gradually over several years. In addition to making lifestyle modifications, the treatment for high cholesterol and blood pressure may also involve medication.

The consequences of diabetes on the nervous system

Since the nerves play a significant role in so many of our physical processes, including movement, digestion, sex, and reproduction, the consequences of diabetes on the nervous system can be severe.

The following symptoms are indicative of nerve injury (neuropathy):

- Hands or feet feeling numb or tingly
- Absence of clitoris or penis arousal
- Excessive sweating or Delayed stomach emptying diagnosis

Neuropathy treatments focus on relieving pain, although prescription medicines including those that reduce blood pressure may also be given to assist delay the onset of the illness.

Diabetes and its effects on digestion

Digestion can be impacted by diabetes in a variety of ways. Constipation, nausea, and diarrhea can result from nerve damage brought on by diabetes.

The side effects of diabetic treatment might also contribute to disrupted digestion.

For example, several drugs for type 2 diabetes might cause digestive problems, though these usually go away as the body gets adjusted to them.

Diabetes and its effects on the skin

Diabetes often affects the skin as a result of its effects on the nerves and circulation, which can result in dry skin, sluggish wounds, burn, and cut healing, fungal and bacterial infections, and loss of sensation in the foot.

It is advised that diabetics get their feet examined at least once a year. Diabetic foot is a term used frequently to describe how diabetes affects the feet.

Fertility and sexual well-being

The body's capacity to send and respond to sexual cues, as well as sexual function, may be negatively impacted by diabetes-related damage to blood vessels and the autonomic nervous system.

Those with diabetes are more than three times as likely to experience erectile dysfunction, and it can manifest 10 to 15 years earlier than in those without the illness.

The influence of diabetes on mental health and concerns that sex might cause hypoglycemia by lowering blood sugar levels are two additional ways that persons with diabetes may have decreased confidence in their sex life.

• confusion over how to use an insulin pump

•the condition's impact on mental health

•worry that sex may lower glucose levels, leading to hypoglycemia.

Chapter 2

Hyperinsulinemia and insulin resistance

When you have more insulin in your blood than is regarded as normal, you have hyperinsulinemia. Your pancreas produces and secretes insulin, a hormone necessary for survival and controlling blood glucose levels, specifically by reducing glucose levels.

The most common cause of hyperinsulinemia is insulin resistance, which occurs when the cells in your muscles, fat, and liver don't react to insulin as they should. In order to keep your blood sugar levels in a safe range, your body produces more insulin (hyperinsulinemia) as insulin resistance progresses.

Hypoglycemia, or low blood sugar, is caused by an overabundance of insulin in a person who does not also have insulin resistance. Excess insulin does not result in low blood sugar when there is hyperinsulinemia brought on by insulin resistance.

Hyperinsulinemia and persistent insulin resistance can cause hyperglycemia, which can develop to Type 2 diabetes and pre-diabetes.

People frequently mix up hyperinsulinemia with hyperinsulinism because of the terms' resemblance. A separate disorder called hyperinsulinism occurs when a person has too much insulin in their blood as a result of a pancreatic problem. This might be an insulinoma, a tumor that overproduces insulin, or a congenital disorder (a disease you have from birth) in which a gene mutation results in excessive insulin production. Low blood sugar results from hyperinsulinism, not hyperinsulinemia.

How typical is hyperinsulinemia?

The simplest approach to gauge the prevalence of hyperinsulinemia is by counting the number of prediabetes cases because there are no routine tests to check for it and no symptoms until insulin resistance progresses to prediabetes or Type 2 diabetes. In the US, more than 84 million persons have pre-diabetes. About one in three adults fall into this category.

Who is affected by hyperinsulinemia?

Anyone can develop hyperinsulinemia due to insulin resistance, and it can be either transient or persistent. Excess body fat, particularly in the abdominal area, and inactivity are the two primary variables that appear to lead to insulin resistance and hyperinsulinemia.

How does my body respond to hyperinsulinemia?

The following conditions are linked to hyperinsulinemia in addition to prediabetes and Type 2 diabetes:

The syndrome is metabolic.

• Overweight.

• PCOS, or polycystic ovarian syndrome.

• Higher levels of triglycerides.

• Elevated uric acid.

• Artery hardening (atherosclerosis).

• Hypertension, or high blood pressure.

Significances and causes

Which signs and symptoms accompany hyperinsulinemia?

You might not exhibit any observable signs of hyperinsulinemia brought on by insulin resistance. This is due to the fact that your pancreas can create enough insulin to go past the resistance. However, pre-diabetes and Type 2 diabetes are frequently brought on by persistent insulin resistance and hyperinsulinemia.

Many people with pre-diabetes go years without showing any symptoms, however, some may have the following signs and symptoms:

• Skin tags, which are tiny skin growths.

• Modifications in the eyes that might cause diabetic retinopathy.

• Acanthosis nigricans, or darkened skin in the armpits or on the back and sides of the neck.

Diabetes type 2 symptoms include:

• Increased thirst.

• Frequently going potty.

• A rise in hunger.

• Cloudy vision.

• Migraines.

• Skin and vaginal infections.

• Wounds and cuts that heal slowly.

If you have any of these symptoms, it's critical that you visit a doctor.

Why does hyperinsulinemia occur?

Hyperinsulinemia is mostly caused by insulin resistance. In order to try to keep your blood sugar levels within a safe range, your pancreas must produce additional insulin since insulin resistance prevents your body from utilizing insulin as it should.

Tests and diagnosis

How is insulin resistance identified?

Since hyperinsulinemia frequently has no symptoms until it causes pre-diabetes or Type 2 diabetes, it can be difficult to detect. Furthermore, since insulin levels can vary greatly during the day, there is no commonly used test to precisely assess elevated insulin levels.

Since there isn't a single test that can accurately identify hyperinsulinemia, your doctor will take a number of things into account while evaluating the condition, including:

• Medical background.

• Ancestral history.

• A medical exam.

• Symptoms and signs.

• The outcomes of blood tests, such as fasting plasma glucose (FPG) test outcomes.

Control and treatment

What's the remedy for hyperinsulinemia?

The main treatment for hyperinsulinemia is lifestyle change because some of the causes of hyperinsulinemia, such as genetics and age, cannot be cured. Changes in lifestyle include:

• Diet: Your doctor or dietitian may advise limiting harmful fat, sugar, red meats, and processed carbs while avoiding consuming excessive amounts of carbohydrates, which trigger excessive insulin production. They'll likely suggest switching to a diet high in whole foods, which includes more fruits, vegetables, whole grains, fish, and lean meat.

Exercise can help cure hyperinsulinemia since it decreases insulin levels and progressively improves insulin sensitivity.

• Weight loss: Losing weight is linked to a reduction in hyperinsulinemia, whereas gaining weight is linked to an increase in hyperinsulinemia. Hyperinsulinemia is improved by treating obesity with dietary changes, lifestyle adjustments, medication, or bariatric surgery.

Within a week following surgery, hyperinsulinemia in class III obese patients who have bariatric surgery is quickly corrected. In addition, between six and 24 months following surgery, insulin sensitivity increases. Bariatric surgery is not appropriate for everyone, though. With your healthcare provider, go through the ideal therapeutic path.

Is it possible to reverse hyperinsulinemia?

There are several causes and contributing factors for insulin resistance, as well as the ensuing hyperinsulinemia. A nutritious diet, frequent exercise, and weight loss are examples of lifestyle improvements that can improve insulin sensitivity while reducing insulin resistance and hyperinsulinemia. However, not all causes can be reversed.

How can you effectively treat insulin resistance and hyperinsulinemia?

Discuss this with your healthcare practitioner.

Prevention

What raises the possibility of hyperinsulinemia?

Your chance of developing hyperinsulinemia is increased by a number of hereditary and lifestyle risk factors. Risk elements include:

• Being overweight or obese, particularly having extra fat around your abdomen.

• Being 45 years or older.

• Having a first-degree family who has diabetes (a biological parent or sibling).

• Leading a physically inactive life.

• Suffering from specific medical disorders, such as high blood pressure or abnormal cholesterol levels.

• A previous heart attack or stroke.

• Having a sleeping condition like sleep apnea.

• Smoking.

Prognosis

What is the outlook (prognosis) for hyperinsulinemia?

The prognosis (outlook) of hyperinsulinemia is influenced by a number of variables, including:

• Insulin resistance's root cause, which results in hyperinsulinemia.

• The degree of hyperinsulinemia and insulin resistance.

• Your propensity for secondary problems brought on by insulin resistance and hyperinsulinemia.

• Treatment adherence and your body's reaction to the medication.

People can have hyperinsulinemia and modest insulin resistance without developing pre-diabetes or Type 2 diabetes. A change in lifestyle can help people with insulin resistance and hyperinsulinemia, both of which are treatable or extremely controllable.

It's critical to control Type 2 diabetes as best you can if hyperinsulinemia leads to the illness in order to avoid potential consequences.

When should I schedule a consultation with my doctor regarding my hyperinsulinemia?

If you have been given a diagnosis of hyperinsulinemia or a disease that is linked to both hyperinsulinemia and insulin resistance, to make sure your blood sugar levels are within a healthy range and that your therapy is functioning, it's crucial to visit your doctor frequently.

Contact your provider if you are exhibiting signs of prediabetes or high blood sugar. To assess your blood sugar levels, they can do quick tests.

Insulin resistance is frequently the cause of the potentially dangerous condition known as hyperinsulinemia. The greatest thing you can do is try to avoid and correct insulin resistance and hyperinsulinemia by keeping a healthy weight, exercising frequently, and eating a nutritious diet because it doesn't have any symptoms until it develops into prediabetes or Type 2 diabetes.

The calorie manipulation in obesity

The notion, which is just that, maintains the idea that you can lose weight by making a daily difference between the calories you eat and burn. Two presumptions exist. According to the first idea, all calories are equivalent, while according to the second, the body handles all calories equally.

We can observe that not all calories are created equal by comparing a Bug Gulp and broccoli. A 7-Eleven Big Gulp has 750 calories and is made entirely of sugar, which equates to 47 teaspoons or one cup. 1.5 tablespoons of naturally occurring sugars are included in the 750-calorie equivalent of broccoli. It would take 21 cups of this vegetable to provide 750 calories.

Chapter 3

How does sugar affect diabetes?

Diabetes of either sort can interfere with the body's capacity to control blood sugar levels.

An autoimmune disorder called type 1 diabetes occurs when the immune system destroys the cells that make insulin. Injuries to these cells compromise the body's capacity to control blood sugar.

When a person has type 2 diabetes, their body's insulin is unable to control the glucose that is released into the blood after eating or drinking.

Consuming excessive amounts of sugar might exacerbate diabetes after it has already developed. Refined carbohydrates like added sugars are easily absorbed into the circulation by the organism. An increase in blood sugar may follow from this.

The body will struggle to transport the glucose in the blood to the body's cells because it either doesn't have enough insulin or can't utilize it properly. Blood glucose levels will continue to be elevated.

Over time, excessive blood sugar levels can harm the body as a whole and lead to diseases including diabetic neuropathy.

Additionally, consuming too many calories might result in weight gain and obesity. One risk factor is obesity.

Which meals and beverages are sugary?

Many foods naturally contain sugars, including fruits and certain vegetables like carrots. Others have sugar that diners may add. People might not realize that many foods have hidden sugars in them.

For instance, 100 grams (g) of ketchup from Trusted Source may include 21.8 g of sugar, which includes glucose, fructose, and maltose. a 12-ounce bottle10 teaspoons of sugar or 160 calories are in a can of soda from Trusted Source. Many processed meals with high sugar content are also deficient in important elements like vitamins and minerals.

Table sugar, usually referred to as sucrose, is a kind of sugar that people add to foods and beverages

• caster sugar for use in baking

• syrup, such as molasses or agave syrup

• honey

• molasses

• cane sugar

• corn sweetener

- high fructose corn syrup

- fruit juice concentrate

Natural sugar-containing foods include:

- fruits and certain vegetables, which contain fructose;

- Lactose-containing dairy products, such as milk

- oatmeal; smoothies and liquids

The following foods include extra (and perhaps concealed) sugars:

- beverages with added sugar, like soda and energy drinks

- confectionery; cakes, cookies, and other baked items; several processed foods, such as ketchup and prepared meals;

- yogurts and milk with added sugar

- Cereals and breakfast bars

- salad dressings; ice cream;

When reading food labels at the grocery, check for more than just the sugar amount.

- sucrose

- glucose

- fructose

- lactose

- maltose

• galactose

Each of them is a form of sugar.

Diabetes patients should see their doctor about how to adjust their daily carbohydrate intake to account for various sugars.

What percentage of your food and beverage contains sugar?

Advice regarding sugar consumption

The American Heart Association (AHA) advises Trusted Source to consume no more than the following amounts of added sugar per day:

For males   : 9 teaspoons or 36 g or 150 calories

For females : 6 teaspoons or 25 g or 100 calories

health Sugar has 4 calories per gram. Reliable Source. A product will have 60 calories if it has 15 grams of sugar in it.

The World Health Organization advises aiming for fewer than 10% of daily total calories to come from sugar.

Other advice for diabetics includes:

• Opting for carbs with a low glycemic index (GI), including whole grains.

• Choose whole fruit over sweetened snacks or drinks, but keep in mind that fruit contains sugar.

• Choosing fiber-rich foods can help control blood sugar levels and offer sustained energy, such as legumes.

• Choose lean meats and healthy fats to stay satisfied for longer and lower your need for sugary snacks.

• Steer clear of processed foods that are lacking in nutrients and often rich in sugar, salt, and bad fats.

• Eat more frequent, smaller meals. Large meals may increase appetite between meals and blood sugar levels, which may encourage unhealthy snacking.

Here are some tasty, healthy meal alternatives for those with diabetes.

further dangers connected to sugar

Although the connection between sugar and type 2 diabetes is unclear, there is little doubt about the connection between sugar and other medical issues.

Health risks associated with a high sugar intake include dependable source

• a high body weight, which increases the risk of heart disease, some cancers, and type 2 diabetes

• tooth decay

• non-alcoholic-related fatty liver disease

• cardiovascular disease

• metabolic syndrome, which encompasses cardiovascular disease, obesity, and type 2 diabetes

According to the National Institutes of Health Trusted Source, high fructose corn syrup (HFCS) can cause issues including heart disease, obesity, diabetes, and non-alcoholic fatty liver disease. A frequent component of processed foods is HFCS.

Due to these factors, some experts have argued for policies that would reduce the quantity of sugar that kids consume, such as modifications to marketing plans and a higher price on sugar-containing goods.

Diabetes dual defects treatment

The discussion includes the therapeutic objectives for people with type 2 diabetes as well as the factors underlying insulin resistance and secretion.

Sulfonylureas aid in the short-term improvement of beta-cell activity, acute insulin response restoration, and glycemic management. Meglitinides, phenylalanine derivatives, and alpha-glucosidase inhibitors may be helpful for elderly patients and other people with normal fasting blood sugar levels and postprandial hyperglycemia, but they are less successful in helping patients with severe fasting hyperglycemia reach their objective HbA1c values. To enhance glycemic control, beta-cell activity, and the lipid profile, metformin and thiazolidinediones work differently on hepatic, muscle, and adipose tissue. Metformin does not have the same effect on free fatty acids as thiazolidinediones. They may enhance glycemic management and the lipid profile when used with sulfonylureas, metformin, or insulin. To reach therapeutic goals, many patients require combination treatment with one or more insulin sensitizers and an insulin secretagogue. When previous treatments fail to keep the patient's HbA1c level below 7.0%, insulin therapy should be started. In order to avoid diabetic complications, this is essential. To lessen insulin resistance and treat the insulin resistance syndrome, insulin sensitizers should be maintained during insulin treatment.

Improvement in glycemic control and the avoidance of diabetic complications are among the therapeutic aims for people with type 2 diabetes mellitus. To lower HbA1c levels and prevent beta cell glucotoxicity, elevated fasting blood sugar levels should be treated before postprandial levels. In order to reduce the elevated cardiovascular risk found in patients with diabetes, which is the primary cause of mortality, dyslipidemia, hypertension, and hypercoagulability should be managed.

Metabolic system

A metabolic syndrome is a group of illnesses that co-occur and raise your risk of type 2 diabetes or cardiovascular disease (heart disease or stroke). Although the causes of metabolic syndrome are complex and unclear, it is thought that a hereditary link exists. Your risk increases if you are physically sedentary and overweight or obese. The terms "metabolic syndrome" and "insulin-resistance syndrome" are sometimes used interchangeably.

As we age, our activity levels tend to decline, and weight gain is a possibility. Since the majority of this weight is in the abdomen, it may lead to the onset of insulin resistance in the body. This indicates that insulin is less efficient throughout the body, notably in the muscles and liver.

Australian individuals over the age of 35 have metabolic syndrome. Patients with diabetes are more prone to develop this.

How to reduce the risk of metabolic syndrome

At least one disorder associated with metabolic syndrome is present in more than half of all Australians. To reduce your risk, consider the following suggestions:

• Implement as many healthy lifestyle changes as you can; a balanced diet, consistent exercise, and weight loss will significantly lower your risk of metabolic syndrome-related illnesses including diabetes and heart disease.

•Change your diet by consuming more natural whole-grain meals, veggies, and fruit. Reduce your meal intake and avoid foods heavy in fat or sugar to aid in weight reduction. Reduce the amount of saturated fats in meat, full-fat dairy, and many processed meals. Stop drinking or limit your consumption to no more than two alcoholic beverages each day.

• Increase your level of physical activity — Depending on what works best for you, regular exercise can take many various forms. Try to exercise for at least 30 minutes each day for at least five days a week. Additionally, try to avoid sitting down for extended periods of time by getting up and taking a one- to two-minute stroll.

•Manage your weight by getting more exercise and adopting healthier eating habits to help you lower your weight.

• Give up smoking. Smoking raises your chances of lung illness, cancer, heart disease, and stroke. Especially if you have metabolic syndrome, quitting will have several positive effects on your health.

• Medication may be indicated - although lifestyle modifications are crucial in the care of metabolic syndrome, medication may occasionally be required to control the various symptoms. To keep their blood pressure and cholesterol within acceptable ranges, some people will need to take antihypertensive drugs to manage high blood pressure or lipid-lowering medications (or both). The most crucial thing is to lower your risk of diabetes, heart attack, and stroke.

•To determine the best management approach for you, speak with your doctor.

Things to keep in mind about metabolic syndrome

• The Metabolic syndrome is a group of illnesses that frequently co-occur and raise your risk of diabetes, heart disease, and stroke.

•Obesity, high blood pressure, high blood triglycerides, low levels of HDL cholesterol, and insulin resistance are the key features of metabolic syndrome. The keys to avoiding or conquering issues associated with metabolic syndrome include healthy food and increased physical activity.

Chapter 4

Type 2 Diabetes and insulin

Insulin is used by around one in four persons with type 2 diabetes. It's not always type 1 Diabetes if you have type 2 diabetes and are administered insulin. You have type 2 diabetes, but your prescription has changed.

Insulin is used as a treatment for type 2 diabetes because the insulin your body produces either does not work as it should, which is known as insulin resistance, or because in some cases insulin resistance causes the pancreas to initially produce more and more insulin to help, but over time the pancreas can become exhausted and start to produce less insulin. It can be necessary to use it as a cure as a result.

It's not your fault if you require insulin as medication, and it doesn't indicate your diabetes hasn't been adequately controlled. It is only another drug that can support your continued good health. And insulin could be the best course of action for you.

When managing type 2 diabetes without insulin, there are six things to be aware of:

When diabetes is more difficult to control at certain points in a person's life, such as during pregnancy, a serious illness, or right after surgery, some individuals may need to take insulin.

When using insulin, it's important to keep up with appointment attendance and to take care of your health. Keeping active and following a healthy diet helps lower your chance of developing diabetic problems.

Weight gain is one of the negative effects of commencing insulin therapy for some people. It might be difficult to manage this on top of finding out you have type 2 diabetes or having your treatment plan changed.

People with type 2 diabetes may occasionally require insulin injections to control their blood sugar levels. Others can manage type 2 diabetes without insulin. Your doctor may advise you to manage type 2 diabetes with a mix of lifestyle modifications, oral drugs, or other therapies, depending on your medical history.

Six things regarding controlling type 2 diabetes without insulin are listed below:

Some persons with type 2 diabetes are able to regulate their blood sugar levels alone by making lifestyle adjustments. But even if you do require medicine, leading a healthy lifestyle is crucial.

Eat a healthy, balanced diet, engage in at least 30 minutes of aerobic activity five days a week, and engage in at least two sessions of muscle-strengthening exercises each week to help control your blood sugar levels.

Your doctor could advise you to lose weight based on your height and current weight. You may create a secure and efficient weight loss strategy with the assistance of your doctor or nutritionist.

It's also critical to abstain from cigarette use to reduce your chance of complications from type 2 diabetes. Your doctor may suggest resources to assist you in quitting smoking if you smoke.

There are many different kinds of oral medications.

Your doctor may recommend oral medicines for type 2 diabetes in addition to lifestyle modifications. Your blood sugar levels may be lowered by them.

For the treatment of type 2 diabetes, a wide range of oral drug classes are available, including:

• alpha-glucosidase inhibitors

• biguanides

• bile acid sequestrants

• dopamine-2 agonists

• DPP-4 inhibitors

• meglitinides

• SGLT2 inhibitors

 sulfonylureas

• TZDs

You could require a mix of oral drugs in some circumstances. Oral combination treatment is the name given to this. To discover a drug regimen that works for you, you might need to experiment with a few different kinds.

Your physician could suggest further injectable medications.

Type 2 diabetes is treated with a variety of injectable medications, not just insulin. Your doctor may occasionally recommend additional injectable drugs.

For instance, it is necessary to inject drugs such as amylin analogs and GLP-1 receptor agonists. Both of these types of drugs help you maintain normal blood sugar levels, especially after meals.

You could need to inject a certain prescription every day or once a week, depending on the drug. Ask your doctor when and how to take any injectable medications they may have prescribed. They can teach you how to properly dispose of used needles and inject medicine.

Surgery for weight loss may be a possibility.

Your doctor can suggest weight reduction surgery to manage type 2 diabetes if your body mass index, a measurement of weight and height, satisfies the requirements for obesity. Bariatric surgery or metabolic surgery are other names for this treatment. Your blood sugar levels can be improved, and it can help reduce your chance of developing diabetes complications.

Multiple diabetic organizations supported weight reduction surgery as a treatment for type 2 diabetes in persons with a BMI of 40 or above in a joint statement released in 2016. For those with a BMI of 35 to 39 and a history of attempting ineffectively to control their blood sugar through lifestyle changes and medication, they also advised weight reduction surgery.

If weight reduction surgery is an option for you, your doctor can help you find out.

The adverse consequences of some therapies

There may be negative effects from various medications, surgeries, and other therapies. Each form of therapy has a different risk of adverse effects.

Discuss the possible advantages and disadvantages of using a new drug with your doctor before you begin taking it. Inquire whether it may interfere with any other vitamins or drugs you use. Additionally, you should disclose to your doctor if you are pregnant or nursing because some drugs are not appropriate for usage during these times.

You run the chance of experiencing complications after surgery, such as an infection at the incision site. Consult your doctor about the potential advantages and disadvantages of any procedure before you have it done. Talk to them about the healing process and the precautions you may take to lower your chance of problems following surgery.

Make an appointment with your doctor if you think you've had treatment-related adverse effects. They can assist in identifying the origin of your symptoms. They may occasionally change your treatment regimen to lessen or eliminate negative effects.

Your medical requirements may alter.

Your health and treatment requirements may alter over time. Your doctor may prescribe insulin if you've had trouble controlling your blood sugar with lifestyle modifications and other drugs. You can better control your disease and reduce your risk of problems by adhering to their recommended treatment schedule.

Oral hypoglycemics

In order to help type 2 diabetic individuals control their disease, oral hypoglycemic medicines are anti-diabetes treatments.

What are Hypoglycemic Agents?

To reduce the amount of glucose in circulation, oral hypoglycemic medications are utilized. These drugs don't really make insulin; instead, they help the pancreas make it. Adult-onset diabetes mellitus, often known as Type 2 or non-insulin dependent diabetes, is typically treated with these medications.

Be aware that while these oral hypoglycemic medications assist manage diabetes, they do not cure it.

An individual with diabetes must be assisted in maintaining normal blood sugar levels by oral hypoglycemic medications in addition to diabetic diet and exercise regimens. The danger of diabetes complications, such as problems with the eyes, heart, kidneys, or blood vessels, is reduced when blood sugar levels are steady. So, that was the definition of an oral hypoglycemic agent. I'll now discuss the several kinds of oral hypoglycemic medications.

The use of oral hypoglycemic drugs

• Sulfonylureas (glipizide, glyburide, gliclazide, glimepiride)

• Meglitinides (repaglinide and nateglinide)

• Biguanides (metformin)

• Thiazolidinediones, including pioglitazone and rosiglitazone

• -Glucosidase inhibitors (voglibose, acarbose, and miglitol)

• Drugs that inhibit DPP-4 such as sitagliptin, saxagliptin, vildagliptin, linagliptin, and alogliptin

• SGLT2 inhibitors (dapagliflozin and canagliflozin)

• Cycloset (bromocriptine)

how to know whether you need insulin

You might not need to start using insulin immediately away after obtaining a type 2 diabetes diagnosis, unless the levels of sugar in your blood are really high. Short-term insulin therapy can help you swiftly lower your blood sugar levels.

But if other drugs haven't helped you regulate your blood sugar levels or aren't right for you, you could also need to start insulin as a therapy.

Chapter 5

Managing gestational Diabetes

A kind of diabetes called gestational diabetes appears during pregnancy and goes away once the baby is born.

Many diabetic drugs have negative interactions with a growing fetus, so a person should ask their doctor about pregnancy-safe substitutes for raising insulin and lowering blood sugar levels.

People with gestational diabetes need to control their sugar consumption and exercise regularly. To assist them control their blood sugar levels, however, if this does not have the intended result, their doctor may prescribe insulin.

There are very few reliable studies that demonstrate which non-insulin drugs are safe to use while pregnant. Although some doctors may prescribe them, the American Diabetcs Association cautions against using them while pregnant.

modifications to lifestyle for type 2 diabetes

Exercise and nutrition are the two key dietary and lifestyle adjustments that can treat type 2 diabetes.

It's crucial to remember, though, that not all people with type 2 diabetes are obese.

Exercise and weight loss

The first stages in treating type 2 diabetes are frequently eating a wholesome, nutrient-dense diet and exercising frequently.

A 2022 consensus statement from the American College of Sports Medicine found that for every kilogram (kg) of body weight reduced, increasing physical activity can cut the risk of type 2 diabetes by 16%.

People with type 2 diabetes are advised by the Centers for Disease Control and Prevention (CDC) Trusted Source to engage in 150 minutes per week of aerobic exercise, which might include:

• brisk walking

• bicycle riding

•swimming

A person can better manage this quantity of exercise by splitting it up into five sessions of 30 minutes each over the week. The body may be able to handle diabetic symptoms with just this.

Diet tips

Dietary advice for controlling type 2 diabetes includes:

• Limiting carbs: Eating more high-protein and high-fiber meals in place of carbohydrates will help control blood sugar.

• Cutting less on sugar: Some people may find that sugar substitutes like stevia can help them control their diabetic symptoms.

• Foods high in fiber: Fiber helps slow down the digestion of sugars and carbs.

Include these foods in your diet:

• vegetables

• fruits

• whole grains

• proteins

• low-fat dairy products

The body gets all the nutrients it needs when the diet is diverse. Additionally, people should strive to consume comparable quantities of carbs at each meal and eat fewer calories overall.

Fish, nuts, and vegetable oils are just a few examples of foods high in polyunsaturated fats that are excellent for regulating blood sugar levels.

A heart-healthy diet, like the DASH diet, can be a very efficient method to design an eating plan to lower the risk or consequences of diabetes Trusted Source.

Surgery

Bariatric surgery can help someone lose weight if lifestyle modifications and exercise are not feasible or effective.

However, this is frequently the final course of action. It is often only prescribed to patients with severe obesity for whom no previous treatments have worked.

In this kind of surgery, the stomach organ is shrunk to make patients feel fuller after eating. Some surgical procedures can also affect a person's anatomy and even their hormone levels, which can lead to weight gain.

Two common instances of this type of medical intervention are gastric band surgery and gastric bypass surgery. Both procedures include dangers, therefore doctors often do not suggest them as a first resort. Bariatric surgery is also seldom covered by insurance companies.

Intermittent fasting

Any dietary plan that alternates between meals and fasting intervals is referred to as intermittent fasting (IF). There are many various kinds of programs, some of which limit calories just during particular times of the day or days of the week. Researchers opted to investigate the effects of a particularly specialized sort of IF diet on those who already have diabetes since this type of diet has become an increasingly popular method of weight loss and has been demonstrated to assist people minimize their risk of heart disease and diabetes.

The intervention group's members did not abstain from food or even restrict when they ate during the day. Instead, they adhered to a certain diet and sometimes limited their calorie intake.

How might intermittent fasting assist in achieving therapeutic objectives? Because of reduced glucose levels and increased insulin sensitivity, IF lowers insulin levels. A person's ability to regulate their weight is aided by the reduced adipose development that results from the lowered insulin level. The prevention of the onset of Type 2 Diabetes Mellitus (T2DM) and the effective management of T2DM are both supported by strong and consistent evidence. Modest weight reduction enhances insulin sensitivity and glycemic control in individuals with T2DM who are overweight or obese and postpones the need for glucose-lowering medications. Dietary energy restriction can produce persistent DM remission for at least two years by significantly lowering HbA1c and fasting glucose. Additionally, a decline in atherosclerosis formation is linked to an increase in insulin sensitivity. This is due to the fact that insulin resistance has the intrinsic propensity to produce atherosclerosis and its problems by increasing C-reactive protein, decreasing LDL particle size, and increasing insulin resistance. Therefore, because it can improve metabolic and inflammatory pathways and lower the likelihood of negative cardiovascular outcomes, intermittent fasting is possibly a viable therapy option. Sutton et al. conducted a cross-over trial in which eight men were randomly assigned to two groups. These men had increased BMI, HbA1c, impaired fasting glucose, and impaired glucose tolerance. OGTT after two hours was 154 mg/dL, the IFG level was 102 mg/dL, and the mean BMI was 32.2 kg/m2. In the first group, participants had a six-hour feeding window that ended at 3 o'clock in the afternoon, whereas the control group got a 12-hour window. The transition to the opposite group took place after five weeks. Individuals in the early time-restriction feeding group had low insulin levels, improved insulin sensitivity and -cell responsiveness, lower blood pressure, and lessen oxidative stress. 70 individuals with metabolic syndrome and a mean BMI of 31.5 kg/m2 participated in a randomized trial by Parvaresh et al., where they were randomly assigned to either a modified ADF or a 25% calorie restriction group for eight weeks. During the three fast days (Saturday, Monday, and Wednesday), patients in the ADF group were instructed to follow an extremely low-calorie diet (75% energy restriction). Then, on the three feed days (Sunday, Tuesday, and Thursday), they consumed a portion of food that met all of their energy requirements. According to the study's findings, the ADF group significantly reduced fasting plasma glucose levels, body weight, waist circumference, and systolic blood pressure more than the group that only restricted calories did. In ten T2DM patients receiving just metformin treatment, observational research demonstrated a reduction in body weight, fasting, and postprandial glucose levels following two weeks of daily fasting for 18–20 hours. According to the research described above, intermittent fasting aids in glycemic goal achievement and weight management, whether or the medication is used. IF has a more profound impact on reaching treatment objectives pre-diabetes and T2DM than simple calorie restriction regimens.

IF's limitations in the treatment of T2DM Medical recommendations on how to manage therapeutic IF in individuals with DM are as few as studies on the safety and advantages of IF with DM. The kind of diabetes medication a person is taking affects the possible hazards that intermittent fasting may bring about, therefore it is important to pay close attention to this information while creating a treatment plan. Anti-diabetic medications with minimal risk of hypoglycemia include metformin, acarbose, thiazolidinediones (TZDs), GLP-1 RAs, and dipeptidyl peptidase-4 (DPP-4) inhibitors. For those who practice intermittent fasting, these medications often don't require dose changes. The potential risk of IF in persons with DM and other comorbidities such as chronic renal disease, chronic liver disease, and heart failure is poorly understood. The risk of hypoglycemia in T2DM patients using insulin or sulfonylureas is known to be elevated. To increase the safety of IF in persons with DM using blood glucose-lowering medications, self-monitoring glucose testing frequency must be increased, or continuous glucose-monitoring devices must be used. Additionally, similar to what might happen in non-diabetic individuals, IF may raise the risk of vitamin and mineral deficiencies as well as protein-energy malnutrition, mostly because current IF regimens place more emphasis on time than content when it comes to calorie intake. In addition, IF increases the risk of developing postural hypotension, gout, peptic ulcers that worsen, irregular menstruation, and cardiac arrhythmias brought on by electrolyte imbalances. The application of IF in the treatment of DM and pre-diabetes requires further research. A healthcare professional should use IF to properly monitor patients, and therapy should be modified in light of the patient's unique circumstances. The maintenance of glycemic goals with monotherapy is frequently only attainable for a few years, after which combination medication is required since T2DM is progressive in many individuals.

Conclusion

Obesity and type 2 Diabetes together make up the "Diabesity" epidemic, which is likely to be the largest in recorded human history. The world can no longer overlook "the rise and rise" of type 2 diabetes, which has been grossly underappreciated as a public health concern. Currently, the IDF Atlas is the source of the majority of national and international diabetes figures. From the standpoint of public health, these estimations have considerable drawbacks. It is clear that the IDF has constantly overestimated the weight of the entire world. There is an urgent need for more accurate projections of the future cost of diabetes. A deeper comprehension of the factors fueling the prevalence of type 2 diabetes is required for prevention. While the "traditional" risk factors for type 2 diabetes, such as heredity, lifestyle, and behavioral changes, have received extensive research for many years, emphasis is now shifting to the influence of the intrauterine environment and epigenetics on future risk in adulthood. It emphasizes the necessity of developing fresh preventative strategies that center on mother and child health. Epigenetic alterations can pass diabetes risk down the generations, feeding a vicious loop that will keep the diabetes pandemic going. The biggest pandemic in human history is, in fact, diabetes. It has had the biggest impact, cost the most money, and is still ongoing.